EATING RIGHT

A Healthy Manual to Overcoming Sickness and Promoting Good Health

By

Charlie Smith

COPYRIGHT

COPYRIGHT©2022 Charlie Smith.

Contents

INTRODUCTION

For some reason, eating healthfully is among the most challenging things a person can accomplish. There are several reasons why eating healthily is challenging, whether due to our lack of resources in many areas or because junk food is readily available.

Yes, we can eat almost anything, and it will keep us alive. We shall be able to function from one moment to the next and claim to be healthy. But is consuming processed meals and sugary beverages as a sole source of nutrition healthy? We should not assume that we are healthy just because we are alive. And as we age, our unhealthy behaviors start to catch up with us more and more.

To avoid any potential problems in the future, it is crucial to establish good eating habits as early as possible. You don't want to discover one day that you've been suffering from a vitamin deficit for years and that it's led to consequences that are nearly impossible to treat. We all need to be more accountable for what we put into our bodies since failing to do so can be pretty damaging.

Of course, hindsight is 20/20 when we are older and can reflect on our errors. We are aware that there were things we could have done and probably should have done but didn't because we were either unaware of the negative consequences or were just lazy. Simply knowing something does not inevitably make the need to act in a health-conscious manner a reality.

Most of the time, it takes being genuinely exposed to the pain that can result from making poor health decisions for us to become more aware of how we handle our bodies and our health in general. Our actions seem more justified when we can't perceive their actual effects.

Remote and challenging to relate to. We might even dismiss them. It can be highly damaging to be in this situation, especially if you are already experiencing the negative impacts of a bad diet and lack of exercise.

Everyone should have the opportunity to grow to their full potential. Still, if we don't even acknowledge the idea that poor eating habits can derail us even in the present, we are eventually saying goodbye to the finest future imaginable. However, anything can change. After reading this book, you will comprehend the significance of eating healthfully and how food affects our bodies and functions.

It can be challenging to stay on track if you don't know why your body responds to food the way it does. But there are several ways you might start to comprehend the significance of consuming healthy meals and how to start on a journey toward healthy eating. Let's stop wasting time now. We should begin to eat well right now!

Chapter 1

Why Eat Healthily

There are several reasons why eating healthily is vital. Most of us are already aware of North America's growing obesity crisis. In general, this is especially true of the United States. The SAD diet is a term that describes the manner that many Americans eat. The term "standard American diet," or "SAD," describes a diet that is deficient in nutrition, has a low intake of vegetables, and is rich in fat and sugar. The SAD diet most likely includes processed foods. These are quick, simple, and readily available foods that have detrimental long-term impacts on health.

Avoiding such processed meals and focusing instead on whole grains, fruits, vegetables, and meat that has not been treated with hormones or other chemicals that may ultimately find their way into your body and create problems is generally regarded as a good option if you want to prevent being obese. Unfortunately, there are many opportunities in North America for us to put off cooking meals.

We have so many items at our disposal, and purchasing poor-quality food costs far less than purchasing high-quality food. It may seem unusual that buying organic costs more than buying foods that may eventually lead to long-term health issues, but supply and demand dictate this.

Additionally, processed foods are mass-produced and highly profitable due to their ease. Because of this, the obesity pandemic in North America is not entirely unexpected. On the list of businesses aiming to profit from people's lack of interest in cooking, nutrition is not at the top.

However, eating well has numerous benefits and compelling arguments against following the typical American diet and processed foods. For instance, you should check into the rest of this book to find strategies to modify your nutrition and start a healthy lifestyle if you do not want to be obese.

By consuming unhealthy foods and adhering to the typical American diet, which is high in fat and sugar, you might increase your risk of contracting diseases. Diabetes is a condition that can arise by eating poorly and is frequently treated with a good diet.

In the end, type II diabetes can be maintained and treated with healthy eating habits and is started by unhealthy eating habits. Make an effort to make wise eating decisions if you want to stay away from these kinds of challenges and issues.

Poor eating can also lead to other ailments. Both chronic illnesses like high blood pressure and others are widespread. Because they didn't make proper food decisions earlier in life, osteoporosis is something that can afflict many people later in life. You can experience cardiac issues, high blood pressure, or poor bone health. All of these put a lot of stress on your body and can be extremely dangerous in the long run.

You should start making decisions that will enable you to stay in their life for as long as possible if you want to demonstrate to your family that you care about them. Your poor health doesn't just affect you. It is something that also has an impact on those close to you. It is rather selfish if people watch you suffer due to your terrible decisions. They are also in pain. Do your best right now to choose what will ultimately be best for your family and yourself. This book will demonstrate how.

Chapter 2

Understanding your relationship with food

Every person gradually starts to form certain habits. In all aspects of our life, we develop habits. We produce various habits related to eating, drinking, working, and personal cleanliness. However, they typically overlook our routines until they start to impact us adversely. Even still, modifying our habits can be very challenging once we realize how negatively our practices affect us. It is like that because that is what I have. Something we do almost subconsciously is called a habit. It requires a lot of willpower to interrupt the pattern because we are hardwired to follow these habits. It becomes much simpler to shift your perspective once you realize that your relationship with food has everything to do with your developed habits and that you can still shape and cultivate.

Your propensity for healthy eating may increase, and your tendency to make decisions that negatively affect you and your future may decrease as you become more aware of the influence and significance of your future and the importance of making positive decisions about these things.

To be honest, many of us think the future is gloomy. We don't perceive compelling enough reasons to alter our behavior because, if there is nothing positive in our future, it doesn't matter whether we make wise decisions. We fail to see how we can genuinely shape the future in a way that serves our interests. Most likely because we don't think we have any control over our lives.

Don't worry if this sensation resonates with you. It is a relatively typical human experience. Because we are frequently instructed what to do by other people, we are typically discouraged from taking control and using our power from a young age and may even cease believing we have any authority over our life.

That makes sense to us as kids. Sometimes kids don't know what's best for them. However, it can foster a mindset of extreme helplessness that makes it difficult for us to see how much our behavior's results can influence who we are and how we show ourselves to others.

This is why it's crucial to genuinely take action to understand better who you are and your eating preferences. When did your routine start? How did you develop that behavior? Why?

What advantages does this behavior give you? What drawbacks does this behavior cause you?

So that you may start to genuinely comprehend how you influence your future with the food you consume, ask yourself as many of these questions as possible. Do you envision a vibrant and healthy future or one that is gloomy and might have many unfavorable health effects?

Next, consider how disciplined you are. Are you able to exercise discipline in making decisions? Or do you have trouble in this area? Everyone can find it challenging to maintain their field, so if you identify with this, you should consider how you can motivate yourself to be physically and psychologically more disciplined.

Then and only then will you indeed be prepared to start your journey toward healthy eating because unhealthy lifestyle choices are prevalent everywhere, whether we like it or not. They are simple and addictive.

It won't matter whether you occasionally consume nutritious food or not if you give in to these bad decisions and don't try to improve your behaviors. The harmful effects will still hold onto your body, ready to emerge when you least expect them. In a sense, unhealthy eating is a habit of self-destructive behavior many of us engage in. Self-destructive eating patterns are risky, whether due to low self-esteem or just because we are unhappy with our lives and lack faith in the future. Before adopting a healthy lifestyle, you must look inward and sincerely respect your life and future. There are numerous ways to accomplish this, and if at all possible, you might want to seek the assistance of a mental health expert. Sometimes they can assist us in seeing biases and negative trends in our life that we are blind to. Once things are recognized and accepted, it may be much simpler to move past them and take the necessary actions to make good decisions.

You can do many things to improve your thinking, whether or not you seek the assistance of a trained expert. You will enable yourself to take the actions required to get there as long as you believe that you are deserving of a healthy body and a bright future. It will be much more difficult if you do not feel good about yourself. You'll be more successful on your trip if you can better grasp your habits, mental barriers, and discipline. Healthy eating is one significant step we can all take every day to become the best versions of ourselves. Additionally, we can do it right now!

CHAPTER 3

THE DANGERS OF DIET TRENDS

Today's society is rife with diet trends, and almost all of them are associated with risks. Sadly, the majority of people who are eager to make money frequently ignore the long-term health effects of their products. Their primary interest is making money, and they are working to build something that will allow them to take advantage of the great need many people have to lose weight quickly and easily. If diet trends are something that piques your attention, there is something that you will have to accept. Unfortunately, there is no suitable technique to lose weight quickly and effortlessly without effort, a nutritious diet, or exercise. If you are overweight or need more mobility due to insufficient fitness, losing weight is a desirable objective.

We can all agree that sometimes we need to start living healthier lives. Instead of putting our trust in businesses that want to take advantage of us to profit, we can do this by eating well and moving our bodies. Some current eating trends are incredibly harmful and have severe short- and long-term health effects. Many rely on techniques that deprive Robert's body and ourselves of vital nutrients—even dehydrating us at times.

These diet fads are abhorrent in every way. They are preying on those who desire health but lack the knowledge to achieve it. They prey on people, frequently women in particular, who are breaking under the weight of unattainable beauty standards and are told that they need to look a certain way to be considered valuable.

That is wholly false. You have worth whether you are 100 or 700 pounds. However, eating healthily is one of the few effective methods you'll be able to jump-start your metabolism and provide your body with the nutrition it needs to operate at its peak potential. When you deprive your body of the vitamins and minerals it needs to survive and rely on a diet fad to educate you on how to slim down and feel good when all they want is your cash, you will find yourself more behind than when you started. The unpleasant reality is that many diet fads send the body into famine mode.

Your metabolism could be damaged by this, which would make you gain weight more quickly in the future. Don't let the advertising that claims to make weight loss quick and simple take advantage of you. All of that will be expensive. Additionally, health fads, like the HCG diet, can seriously mess with your body and hormones.

Diet trends are hilarious in that they frequently lead to unhealthy and challenging methods of weight maintenance, which will make it more difficult for you to lose weight in the future. Do not believe a drug you see advertised on television if you want to lose weight. Replace unhealthily processed and sugary foods with whole-grain alternatives and organic fruits and vegetables to avoid introducing chemicals into your body that will make it more difficult for you to lose weight and ultimately disrupt your body chemistry. It may be alluring to lose weight rapidly without giving up the unhealthy eating habits you have accumulated over the years, but this is unhealthy. If you are not careful about how you try to reduce weight, you are harming yourself and setting up your body for future health issues. Aim to make decisions you want others to make for themselves by doing everything you can. Before you succumb to the TV snake oil salesman, do some homework. Look into these issues because you deserve to do things correctly and don't want your future muddled by the negative repercussions of a sales pitch that cares about your wallet and not your well-being.

CHAPTER 4

THE FOOD PYRAMID

The food pyramid has most likely been seen by all of us. We frequently utilized the food pyramid as a guide while growing up to give us an idea of how much and what kind of food we should eat each day to maintain a healthy lifestyle.

Of course, there is always proof that the food pyramid is flexible, but overall, if you can follow the food pyramid, you'll have a rough understanding of what constitutes a balanced, healthy diet. Even if this is occasionally debatable, eating some staples is nevertheless beneficial. Maybe one that you come up with yourself. Many assert that eating as many grains as the food pyramid may have recommended is no longer considered the healthiest course of action. Many people are promoting a no-grain lifestyle as the healthiest option in light of recent celiac disease outbreaks.

Try to evaluate your unique experiences with food before depending on the food pyramid as your fundamental guideline for what is healthy to consume. With a lot of grains, some people are healthier, while others are not. To the best of your

ability, use your judgment in this situation so that you can move in the appropriate way for your health.

The traditional food pyramid suggests the following:

1. Up to 11 servings of bread, pasta, cereal, and rice can be consumed daily.
2. You need three to five servings of fruits and vegetables daily.
3. If you are not allergic to anything or lactose intolerant, you are permitted to have two or three servings of their eggs every day.
4. Eating two or three portions of meat and beans daily and other foods like nuts, fish, and chicken are advised.
5. Unsurprisingly, the top list comprises items like sugar, fat, and oil. Because you shouldn't have too much of any of these; instead, utilize them sparingly to ensure you lead the healthiest lifestyle possible.

Once more, this is merely a reference to the conventional food pyramid. You may need to alter this chart to suit your particular needs and dietary requirements. This is the norm for the food pyramid. However, that can be used to your absolute advantage to develop a healthier lifestyle if you do not have any particular needs.

CHAPTER 5

HOW FOOD CAN BE YOUR MEDICINE

In the same way that eating poorly can make you unwell, eating well can frequently make you feel better and help you recover from illness.

Additionally, it can be used as a defense against disease. In truth, Ayurveda, a comprehensive healing system, has been practiced in India for thousands of years.

This age-old treatment method treats any condition by altering your diet. The food that has kept Indians alive for many years is their medication. And it might still be relevant today. Many cures are nothing more than wholesome meals with anti-inflammatory characteristics and the capacity to nourish your body from the inside out. Healthy food choices have been shown to impact anything from cancer to infections. And that has never been clearer than with this traditional healing technique.

However, a lot of it has been tried and true for thousands of years and will continue to impact the body. Of course, much of modern technology will disapprove of these methods because they have not been scientifically investigated.

Food can ultimately determine whether or not you are susceptible to illness and whether or not you believe in the ancient healing art. Your body will be stronger and more capable of fighting disease and infection if you eat well than if you are undernourished and following the typical American diet.

Fighting off the unpleasant consequences of the disease can be nearly impossible if your body lacks the necessary vitamins and minerals.

It may occasionally even result in disease. Certain types of poor unprocessed foods might cause illnesses and increase your risk of developing certain cancers if you eat them often.

There are numerous examples of people who could live long and healthy lives merely by changing the way they needed, even though cancer is still being investigated and has not yet been fully understood by the scientific world well enough to be cured. A healthy diet can aid in reducing the symptoms of numerous ailments that are difficult and incurable, such as multiple sclerosis.

They will continue to do this as long as you ensure that everything you put into your body nourishes and gives your organs and cells all the fuel and resources required to keep your body strong. And they'll try their hardest to succeed.

However, if you are deliberately harming your body, it won't be able to fight back as well as it could if it were well nourished. Because of this, you must pay attention to how you feed your body. You may be setting yourself up for failure in ways that you may later come to regret if you are not actively and consciously choosing the food that you consume.

CHAPTER 6

THE HEALTH BENEFITS OF EATING VEGETABLES

Especially when it comes to the typical American diet, vegetables are one of the world's most underrated foods. Most people are unaware of how crucial it is to give the body the vitamins and minerals only veggies can offer. People occasionally consider veggies to enhance their beauty, but when it comes to improving their health, they tend to lose interest.

However, it is safe to presume that you are willing and able to evaluate why it is vital to consume veggies now that you are here and reading this book. Here are some of the finest justifications for regularly including vegetables in your diet.

First and foremost, fiber is necessary for the body to eliminate extra waste. If there is no method to move the trash out of the body and stop it, it can cause weight gain and other problems by remaining inside the body.

There are other benefits to fiber as well. It can assist you in lowering your risk of developing heart disease and help you stop your blood cholesterol from rising. Vegetables contain folic acid, which is also present there and can help your body produce red blood cells if you consume enough of it. This can be quite helpful in preventing anemia and can be especially advantageous to women, who tend to need this ingredient during pregnancy and menstruation.

Several vitamins, including vitamins A and C, which aid in preventing illness and maintaining bodily health, are naturally abundant in vegetables. In addition to assisting in the fight against and prevention of anemia, it can help you heal more quickly and absorb iron. Potassium is abundant in vitamins, which is beneficial since it keeps the body from developing high blood pressure. It has been demonstrated that eating vegetables lowers the incidence of stroke and other heart-related issues. They can stop the formation of kidney stones and the breakdown of bone tissue. Vegetables are an excellent strategy to help you control type II diabetes and obesity.

Additionally, it can support your resilience in the fight against cancer and cancer prevention. Vegetables are shallow in fat and have external calorie content, possibly one of their best attributes. This implies that you don't need to worry too much about putting on weight if you eat as many vegetables as you like. You can lessen hunger pangs and maintain focus on a healthy lifestyle by snacking on vegetables.

Vegetables have so many beautiful qualities. The fact that they are so uncommon in the typical American diet is unexpected. Walking outside your grocery store first is one of the best strategies to assist yourself avoiding processed goods that are heavy in fat, sugar, and salt.

Instead of skipping to the finish and cheating by choosing pasta and other processed foods that are poor in nutritional vegetable content, proceed through the fresh produce department to make deliberate selections to give your body healthy new vegetable options. Making decisions that will fuel your body is the first step in healthy eating, and few foods are nourishing than veggies.

Because of early unhealthy and poor eating habits or even self-imposed later in life, we might frequently lose our taste for healthy meals, but it is simple to get back on track. Give vegetables some space in your schedule. The advantages may be worth the extra time it takes to prepare them.

CHAPTER 7

THE HEALTH BENEFITS OF EATING FRUITS

Unfortunately, it is well-known that those who consume the typical American diet do not consume enough fruit. The fruit they consume is typically found in cans or heavily sweetened. Fruit with added sugar cancels out any health advantages that consuming fruit in its natural state can have for the body.

Overeating fruit might have certain drawbacks, especially if you have diabetes. The fruit has many naturally occurring sugars and juicing yields a lot of sugar without a lot of fiber, which might give the body an excess. Fruit's high fiber content, which lowers heart disease risk and prevents constipation, is one of its nutritional qualities. Additionally, meals high in fiber, such as fruits and vegetables, are excellent for managing weight because they make you feel full on fewer calories. Fruit also contains many vitamins and minerals, especially vitamin C, which is particularly abundant in citrus fruits.

Vitamin C is a force to be reckoned with when promoting the body's healing ability. Vitamin C-rich fruits will do the trick if you want something to keep your teeth and gums healthy. Fruit can also aid the body in preventing kidney stones and strokes, two different goals. Fruits strengthen the body and aid in preventing and treating diseases like skin illnesses and heart issues. When trying to eliminate destructive items from your diet, fruit can be one of the healthiest methods to boost energy and satisfy any sugar cravings you may have.

Suppose you are prepared to use the incredible power of fruit. In that case, you may have a nutritious snack that fulfills your sweet desire as long as you aren't going overboard with your fruit intake, such as putting a lot of them in the blender and ultimately consuming excessive sugar.

Both fruits and vegetables have a natural propensity to help your skin glow and appear much more hydrated and nourished if you are interested in the health benefits that food can have. Fruits and vegetables are rich in vitamins, minerals, and antioxidants that give your body the water it needs to maintain healthy skin and look.

It can maintain your skin's youthful appearance and help your hair grow softer and more healthily. By moisturizing your skin and keeping your body clear of waste materials that leak out of your pores, fruit can even help you halt acne in its tracks.

Fruit's high water content is ideal for keeping the body hydrated, and you will see the advantages immediately.

Fruit is also highly beneficial for digestion. It helps to bind waste and aid the body in getting rid of substances that would otherwise cause problems because of the high fiber content. Fruits and vegetables can therefore help with weight loss. The body removes waste before it has a chance to be broken down and stored as fat.

Fruit is another excellent technique for disease prevention and treatment, including cancer. Apples are one fruit that helps prevent asthma attacks. Others have a solid cholesterol-lowering effect.

In particular, red-skinned grapes have a history of being used to treat cancer. They also aid in the treatment of renal and eye conditions. Berries are very beneficial if you have an infection. They contain lots of antioxidants.

Just ensure the produce you consume has not been exposed to industrial pesticides, as doing so could result in problems with your health and the complexity of weight loss.

You can even consume dry fruits to replace unhealthy and sugary snacks and give your body a sweet treat that will be incredibly nutrient-dense. Simply be aware of the sugar content in dried fruits because, occasionally, when offered commercially, extra sugars turn what could be a nutritious pleasure into something that may ultimately contribute to weight gain.

Fruit can, however, assist you in weight loss if you consume it regularly and healthily. Fruit's fibers and water content will fuel your cells and organs while also making your body feel complete as long as you are not overeating foods with a lot of sugar. You can eliminate problems causing obesity thanks to the fibers and water content, and you'll notice a significant improvement in your energy levels overall.

You can use this vigor to work harder at leading a healthy lifestyle and exercise. This might be especially useful if you continue your move toward improved health and well-being by substituting healthy fruit options for sugary junk food.

CHAPTER 8

THE BEST MEAT TO EAT FOR HEALTHY LIVING

Although meat is typically seen as one of the main staple items in an email, you might be surprised to learn that some meats are healthier than others. Of course, we know the distinction between red and white meats. White meats are thought to be leaner and generally more nutritious than red meats, which are more frequently associated with health difficulties and cardiovascular disorders.

Some people might be surprised to learn that other factors contribute to the unhealthiness of meat. Issues include what the animals are given while they are still alive and possible injections of antibiotics and hormones, at least in the case of cows, to help them grow faster or produce more milk.

These hormones eventually find their way into the meat we eat and may negatively affect our health. If we are not careful about the decisions, we make when selecting our foods, they may eventually contribute to future poor health, including but not limited to malignancies and hormone changes that can be very debilitating. However, you will already be ahead of the game if you are confident that the meat you eat comes from reliable suppliers that do not overfeed animals with steroids and antibiotics. If not, attempt to find local establishments where you can get beef free of harmful industrial standards by doing some study.

Nevertheless, some meats are healthier than others, even when considering the healthy meat selections. Fish is one of the healthiest meats you can eat, particularly if you're trying to reduce weight. Fish is nutrient-dense and lean. However, you need to be cautious about where your fish comes from.

While some fish may come from regions where mercury contamination is possible, other fish may be grown in unhygienic settings. For this reason, it is unwise for pregnant women to consume fish or shellfish.

But if you can discover a good source of fish, your body can benefit greatly from this. Omega-3 fatty acids, abundant in fish, benefits memory and brain health. Overall, omega-three fatty acids are highly prized, and the body requires them to perform at their best, particularly when it comes to academic affairs. Another excellent choice is chicken, which has been produced in a humane setting. Protein is abundant in chicken.

In actuality, it contains the most protein of any type of meat. They are typically fed meals that won't harm humans' bodies in the same way as eating a lot of beef can, or they are raised in decent conditions.

However, eating grass-fed beef from a reliable source might also be a fantastic alternative. There are typically fewer chances of these animals being raised with harmful carcinogens if you choose to eat organic chicken.

Conventionally raised hens are frequently offered substances that speed up their growth, which can negatively affect the chickens and the people who eat them. They also receive copious amounts of painkillers, antidepressants, and occasionally arsenic and caffeine. Consuming a lot of meat from conventional farms is risky, but if you can locate a reliable provider, you should do it.

Due to its high selenium content, turkey is another excellent meat. This is significantly beneficial to the body as it can aid in removing free radicals and other toxins.

Again, though, you should make an effort to ensure that your meat comes from reliable sources because, in the case of conventionally grown chicken and turkey, it is standard practice to treat them similarly and to feed them harmful chemicals that unnaturally accelerate their rate of growth and ultimately contaminate human bodies with those chemicals.

As long as you avoid eating meat raised using risky or conventional ways, eating meat can be highly healthy for your body overall. These animals are frequently exposed to extremely hazardous substances by both the animals and the people who consume them. It is better to avoid any chemicals that can land in your body and hinder weight loss if you want to eat healthily and lose weight.

Eating healthfully involves staying away from anything that can be harmful to the body, such as hormones and chemicals that might upset our delicate systems, even if you are not trying to lose weight. Fortunately, you can find lean meats from various sources, whether you choose to indulge in chicken, beef, or lamb. There are ways to obtain responsibly farmed, wholesome meat to save your cravings.

CHAPTER 9

THE DANGERS OF PROCESSED FOODS

Nobody is surprised by the fact that processed foods are harmful. However, it is surprising that they are still permitted to be kept on the shelves despite the damage they cause to our bodies and minds. For some people, consuming unhealthy food goes beyond simple personal preference. Because processed foods are a convenient and affordable way to feed large families on a tight budget, people in poverty are occasionally forced to turn to them because of how the economy operates.

The tricky part about it is that over time, these meals lead to medical issues that cost much more money than it would feed a large family with healthy, sustainable options. In the end, it appears that those with little funds suffer in both scenarios.

Foods that have been processed are just unhealthy, even if you don't have to feed a family on a tight budget. Their high fat and sugar content is a contributing factor to why they are so addictive.

They frequently consist of boxed dinners with pasta and a disproportionate amount of sugar. Too much sugar is harmful to those predisposed to type II diabetes. Consuming sugar in large quantities will eventually overload your body, increasing the likelihood that you'll gain weight and experience other health problems.

Because sugar increases insulin resistance, which makes it more challenging, if not impossible, to control your blood sugar levels, sugar cane hasten the development of diabetes.

There will inevitably be a bad outcome if you consume things like these excessively, such as at every meal or every day. Ingesting that much fat and sugar regularly can cause heart disease, cancer, diabetes, and obesity, in addition to the more well-known conditions of obesity and diabetes. This is extremely risky, and processed meals are to be avoided at all costs.

Eating processed foods poses another risk due to their high artificial content and addiction potential. The majority of the foods' constituents do not generally nourish the body. Instead, they make us feel full while depriving our bodies of the necessary nutrients for regular operations.

We ultimately allow ourselves to be dumped down when we consume bland, unnourishing foods. We are not operating at our optimum efficiency level because we are not moving, thinking, or thinking clearly. These activities can cause a lack of coordination, even despair, and are harmful.

We all understand, at some level, those processed meals are less healthy than the kinds of things we ought to be frequently eating. Even though our minds are unaware of it, our bodies are aware. We pay the price for it. We're anxious about it.

Whether or not we are addicted to unhealthy foods, our bodies are aware of when we overindulge. And whether it happens unconsciously or not, we frequently punish ourselves. We are aware that we are misbehaving. Although we are still processing it, we nevertheless feel irritated and dissatisfied.

Artificial colorings, carcinogenic, are also widely used in processed foods. We essentially ingest dye when we consume foods that have a fixed color. Would you desire to consume hair dye? Actually, no. However, these kinds of chemicals are present in your diet. They do not leave your body; they remain there. Your internal organs are colored. They can cause cancer and are quite harmful.

It was additionally loaded with preservatives. Food that has been processed spends a very long period on the shelf. Longer than is advisable or typical. A regular milk bottle can't survive for months on end. It would sour and curdle. The same is true for cheeses and other readily available items with a long shelf life.

Establishing shelf lives is crucial for businesses since they may generate more revenue if their food has a longer shelf life. To make the most significant money possible, they will do whatever it takes, regardless of whether it is better for the human body.

Preservatives frequently contain harmful, synthetic compounds as well as excessive levels of salt. Both of which are completely bad for the body. Because of the high salt content of processed foods, these foods might cause hypertension and heart problems. People who live solely off of processed foods frequently experience high blood pressure, and heart attacks and obesity are among North America's leading causes of death.

Everything in this relates to the typical American diet. The terrible thing is that these processed foods are incredibly addictive even if you know they are bad for you due to the chemicals and excessive sugar and fat content.

The condition can be nearly as harmful as a drug addiction since the body starts to want them. It can have long-term effects on your health and development when you become addicted to a food that is neither nourishing nor healthful.

We absorb processed foods far more quickly than foods high in beneficial dietary fiber, which is another way that they lead to obesity. We may not even be expending as much energy as we would when digesting nutritious foods if we are digesting these foods quickly, and they do not fill us up because we are not getting the fiber that makes us feel full.

As a result, we consume more and digest less, which causes a quick weight gain. When you eat many processed foods, your body contains far more calories. You burn many more calories when you consume wholesome, high-dietary fiber foods.

Unfortunately, this means that whether they want to or not, people who eat a diet high in processed foods will eventually acquire weight. And because they are not nutritional, they won't provide you with the same energy level. Because you consume many more harmful, sugar-filled foods without feeling satisfied or exhausted, they are likely to make you feel sluggish, sleepy, and too full.

Our bodies do not adequately digest processed food. They become fat quite soon. Additionally, they contain a lot of fat. They frequently contain hidden carbohydrates and fats. One of the main ingredients in many of these processed foods is vegetable oil, which is also often combined with high fructose corn syrup, a significant cause of weight gain.

It makes sense that North America is dealing with the worst obesity pandemic in the planet's history if every processed food on the shelves contains high fructose corn syrup, which is valid for most of them. Because they do not degrade, hydrogenated oils are very unhealthy.

They continue to exist in your body and combine with the fat cells. These oils make it much harder to burn off fat. They are more challenging to lose, and this resistant fat can swiftly result in obesity. Most of the nutrients that humans require to function at their best are not present in the ingredients of processed foods. Before completely thriving, we need the fibers, vitamins, and minerals found in natural food.

If you can't avoid eating processed foods, at least consume them in moderation. They pose a threat. They may cause us to feel lethargic, angry, and generally miserable.

When we switch from a healthy diet and eat only processed foods that are too sugary, too fatty, and too unhealthy, our moods can change from good to bad.

Our bodies yearn for food. Giving your body that nutrition is the best and simplest thing you can do for yourself. It can be challenging to adjust to new routines, such as relying exclusively on processed foods, and it can be highly stressful sometimes.

You have to spend much more time in the kitchen preparing meals and caring for your health. However, consuming manufactured foods is ultimately something that can kill you and separate you from who you are. Instead of allowing your body to get rid of the garbage you are putting into it, you are absorbing poisons and avoiding nutrients that can act as antioxidants.

Junk food is the same as processed food. They are the same. They are junk foods that appear healthier. They have merely disguised munchies. Avoiding processed meals at all costs is the first and most effective action you can take to become healthy and genuinely feel well. Do not believe the promises on the package that these foods are healthful.

They lack anything that nourishes your body and are saturated, fat, sugary, and salty. Make every effort to break the habit of relying solely on processed meals. If you put your mind to it, eating healthily is simple and doable.

Just keep in mind to avoid the aisles full of hazardous and seductive packaging that conceals the hazards of the processed food inside by going around the grocery store to pick up the fresh produce and meat.

Chapter 10

Bringing it all together with meal planning

One of the most crucial elements of creating a healthy lifestyle is meal planning. It can be pretty simple to give in to the temptations of the unhealthy meals to which we have grown accustomed when we cannot see the future of our diet. Mainly if we regularly eat them instead of the items that will nourish us.

Planning meals is a big task. It could seem a little scary, particularly to someone who struggles with organizing. Don't worry if you find that organizing your meals is difficult. Whether you lack creativity in the kitchen or not, there are numerous simple and enjoyable ways for you to start preparing your meals.

You can buy a variety of meal planning kits. Many of them allow you to order boxes filled with fresh ingredients and useable recipes for cooking. If you are not accustomed to cooking, as is frequently the case, this can be pretty beneficial.

Especially when it seems challenging to carve out the time necessary to prepare substantial, nutritional meals due to poor eating habits and a hectic work schedule. Research is the first stage in meal preparation. You must consider your options if you want to become healthier.

The most significant first step is to do some recipe research. Building up a binder of nutritious foods you wish to try can be entertaining and enlightening. It might even teach you stuff you didn't know before or open your eyes to various culinary options you might have previously laughed off as being too harsh for you to make.

Recipes have the power to open your mind. Especially if you're eager to learn something new, it can be challenging to develop the habit of cooking, but once you do, you'll be astonished at how much freedom you'll have when putting together a great and healthy meal for yourself!

Look through cookbooks and publications to collect recipes that you wish to try. Start with the foods that appear to be the most delicious and nourishing, and if you are a rookie cook, you might also want to start with the foods that appear to be the most straightforward.

Next, make sure your recipe organization is straightforward and user-friendly. Meal planning will be significantly more challenging if you become disorganized and overwhelmed.

Making sure everything is as simple as possible is essential when starting a new habit. Your system can become overworked if you make too many adjustments at once, so you should always aim to start small and make them easier to maintain until they become second nature.

Ensure they are nearby so you can quickly start preparing your supper when the time comes. If you are using a binder, you might want to laminate the pages or plastic sleeves so that they won't be harmed by water or other food contamination if you use it in the kitchen.

It would be beneficial to arrange your recipes in the following order: breakfast, lunch, supper, and snacks. Once you start cooking, you'll be able to refer to the appropriate recipes with less difficulty. If you'd like, you could even arrange your binder according to the days of the week, with daily meal plans put out in the binder.

Your recipes could be organized in a variety of ways. Follow your intuition and do what seems to make the most sense.

Avoid forcing yourself to follow a system of organizing that is not effective for you. Instead, ensure that you carry out your best course of action.

To keep your creative juices flowing and your kitchen exciting, set aside time each week to look for new recipes that stand out to you. You can try various dishes, and the more you do, the more enjoyable your journey toward healthy eating might be!

Next, look into Microsoft Office programs like Excel to help you manage your meal planning. You can choose from a wide variety of templates in Excel to help you organize your meals by day, time, and week. This could be a handy tool!

You can download apps on your phone, tablet, or another device to help you better use your time and resources if you'd prefer not to use Excel.

Even more traditionally, you can get a notepad made specifically for preparing meals. Organizing and making your meals accessible begins with this crucial step.

When starting a path toward healthy eating, having a meal plan is quite beneficial. It takes time and perseverance to develop excellent habits, and you will inevitably mess up at some point.

However, that does not obligate you to remain rooted to the earth. It implies that you must get back up and continue your efforts because giving up are far simpler than sticking to your original plans.

Sticking with the theme is one strategy that may be incredibly helpful in meal planning. For instance, many people have particular pieces, such as Taco Tuesday or another day that is designated for a specific kind of dish. Feel free to copy that meal planning style if you believe it would help you stay on track. It is done for a reason—it works and keeps things straightforward and efficient.

If you want to things simple that can be an intelligent approach because have to do a lot of planning and preparing every week or month can be annoying. You may alternate between two themes for your biweekly meals: rice and veggies on Tuesday one week and tacos on Tuesday the following. Meal planning can be done in any method. Following through is something you must make sure you do.

Everything else becomes unnecessary and challenging without follow-through. Accountability is a quality that can aid in meal planning success. Ask them whether they would be willing to assist you and stick to your schedule if you told someone who knows you and cares about you that you are trying to organize your meals.

They can assist you by enquiring about your progress and whether you remain on course. Additionally, they can decide to support you and cheer you on in your achievements.

They can be incredibly gratifying for both of you. However, they decide to assist you. It can be wonderful to have people in your corner who genuinely want you to succeed, provided they are good and encouraging. Just make sure you are eliminating toxic individuals who focus on themselves or give you the impression that it will be challenging for you to achieve your objectives.

Sure, receiving constructive criticism can be tremendously helpful, but it can occasionally be toxic if you are not looking for it. Make sure you know the difference between a supportive individual who merely wants to see you succeed and a poisonous person disguising them as encouraging.

Personal accountability is a different way to accept responsibility. Journaling and self-affirmations are practical tools for achieving personal accountability. You may stay focused and check in to see if you are doing the actions you want to take by talking to yourself about your goals, whether you do it privately or aloud.

Instead of criticizing yourself if you discover that you are not, consider your barriers and continue as you start to identify them. If you don't attempt, you'll never succeed in anything. If you make an effort and make positive changes in your life, everything will eventually fall into place.

There are numerous benefits to journaling. They can assist you in remembering what, when, and how much you've eaten. This will help you determine what you may reasonably anticipate from yourself. You should address and note the things that make you miserable. However, remember that it is a process, and you need to move carefully rather than getting frustrated with yourself for not being a trickle right away.

Start slowly by easing into one or two meals a week, and then gradually add in the rest as you feel comfortable with the process, rather than imposing a whole shift in routine and planning for every meal for the next month when you have never done it before.

Make it something that won't startle you. The most durable change is gradual change. And writing in a notebook about your experiences will help you explore your deepest feelings about the procedure and any barriers you didn't even know you had.

You'll start to notice trends in your behavior and maybe even forecast when and why you might be tempted to veer off course. It will be simpler to prevent these trigger points in the future if you recognize them.

It may be a lot of fun and thrilling to arrange meals. It may be pretty satisfying to consider precisely what you will be putting in your body and take the required measures to do so, even if you do not appreciate that type of organization. You will be well on your way to a lifestyle of healthy eating with meal planning and a healthy dose of self-esteem. Everyone deserves the chance to become the most beneficial and fittest version of them possible.

CONCLUSION

It can be challenging to start eating healthily, especially if you were unable to form healthy eating habits as a young child. It is feasible to develop a stronger sense of health awareness and proactively.

Fortunately, we can start improving ourselves and moving forward in life every single day that we wake up breathing.

Being the best version of ourselves can first seem scary, but as you begin to understand that every decision you make affects your life—whether positively or negatively—it gets much simpler to see where our actions are going before they come back to bite us. Poor dietary decisions will undoubtedly haunt us in the future. If we are careless about what we put into our bodies while we are younger, we risk starting to experience health issues later in life. Good food and exercise is the only way to cultivate a healthy and happy body and mind.

When we are confined to our houses all day, consuming only processed meals high in sugar and fat, and sitting around watching TV without exercising, we start to get restless and stir crazy. People are losing their lives as a result of the risky American diet. Don't allow yourself to turn into one of them.

Make the decisions you need to improve yourself and develop into the best version of yourself instead. Make decisions that honor your family and ensure they can count on you for many years.

This is genuinely very selfish when we don't look after ourselves. Whether we are aware of it or not, there are individuals in our immediate vicinity who genuinely care about the people we are and the value we add to their lives. Everyone should be able to shape their future and make decisions that will help them for many years.

One approach to start bettering yourself and preparing your body and mind for the future is through healthy nutrition. You should start eating healthy as soon as possible if you want to be independent and active for as long as you can without spending thousands upon thousands of dollars on medical bills and other expenses.

If not, it will inevitably become a financial and physical burden on your life. You've read this book and used the information in it, so you're better equipped to start living a healthy lifestyle.

Your quality of life will be significantly improved now and in the future if you plan your meals and learn more about why it is crucial to make healthy food choices. The benefits of healthy eating will become apparent as soon as you maintain your commitment! You only need to try. You are capable of completing this.